MedicalCe

The Key Facts on Arthritis

Everything You Need to Know About Arthritis and Rheumatic Diseases

By Patrick W. Nee

www.MedicalCenter.com

Published by:

MedicalCenter.com

96 Walter Street/ Suite 200

Boston, MA 02131, USA

Tel: 617-354-7722

www.MedicalCenter.com

manager@medicalcenter.com

Table of Contents

Chapter 1: Introduction to Arthritis and Rheumatic Diseases

Rheumatoid arthritis is a disease that affects the joints. It causes pain, swelling, and stiffness. If one knee or hand has rheumatoid arthritis, usually the other does too. This disease often occurs in more than one joint and can affect any joint in the body. People with this disease may feel sick and tired, and they sometimes get fevers.

Some people have this disease for only a few months or a year or two. Then it goes away without causing damage. Other people have times when the symptoms get worse (flares), and times when they get better (remissions). Others have a severe form of the disease that can last for many years or a lifetime. This form of the disease can cause serious joint damage.

Who Gets Rheumatoid Arthritis?

Anyone can get this disease, though it occurs more often in women. Rheumatoid arthritis often starts in middle age and is most common in older people. But children and young adults can also get it.

What Causes Rheumatoid Arthritis?

Doctors don't know the exact cause of rheumatoid arthritis. They know that with this arthritis, a person's immune system attacks his or her own body tissues. Researchers are learning many things about why and how this happens. Things that may cause rheumatoid arthritis are genes (passed from parent to child), environment, and hormones.

How is Rheumatoid Arthritis Diagnosed?

People can go to a family doctor or rheumatologist to be diagnosed. A rheumatologist is a doctor who helps people with problems in the joints, bones, and muscles. Rheumatoid arthritis can be hard to diagnose because not only is there no single test for the disease, but the systems can be the same as other kinds of joint disease and the full symptoms can take time to develop.

Ideally, RA is diagnosed early -- within 6 months of symptom onset -- so that treatment can begin as soon as possible to slow or halt disease progression. Early diagnosis is challenging because the symptoms of early RA can be non-specific (e.g., malaise, fatigue, weakness, muscle soreness, low-grade fever, weight loss) and may actually be symptoms of other conditions.

To diagnose rheumatoid arthritis, doctors use medical history, physical exam, x rays, and lab tests.

How is Rheumatoid Arthritis Treated?

Doctors have many ways to treat this disease. The goals of treatment are to take away pain, reduce swelling, slow down or stop joint damage, help people feel better, and help people stay active.

Treatment can include patient education, self-management programs, and support groups that help people learn about treatments, how to exercise and relax, how to talk with their doctor, and problem solving.

These programs help people learn about the disease, reduce pain, cope with physical issues and emotions, feel more control over the disease, build confidence, and most importantly, lead full and active lives.

Treatment for rheumatoid arthritis may involve lifestyle changes, medication, surgery, regular doctor visits, and alternative therapies.

Lifestyle Changes

Some ways to take care of yourself include: keeping a good balance between rest and exercise, taking care of your joints, lowering your stress, and eating a healthy diet.

Medicine

Most people with rheumatoid arthritis take medicine. Drugs can be used for pain relief, to reduce swelling, and to stop the disease from getting worse. What a doctor prescribes depends on one's general health, how serious the rheumatoid arthritis is, how serious the rheumatoid arthritis may become, how long one will take the drug, how well the drug works, and possible side effects that come with taking the drug.

Surgery

There are many kinds of surgery for people with severe joint damage. Surgery is used to reduce pain, help joints work better, and help people resume and accomplish daily activities.

Surgery is not for everyone. Talk about the option with your doctor.

Regular Doctor Visits

Regular medical care is important so doctors can see if the disease is getting worse, see if drugs are helping, look for drug side effects, and change treatment when needed.

Your care may include blood, urine, and other lab tests and x rays.

Alternative Therapies

Special diets, vitamins, and other alternative therapies are sometimes suggested to treat rheumatoid arthritis. Some therapies help people reduce stress. Many of these treatments are not harmful, but they may not be well tested or have any real benefits.

People should talk with their doctor before starting an alternative therapy. If the doctor feels the therapy might help and isn't harmful, it can become part of regular care.

WHAT RESEARCH IS BEING DONE ON RHEUMATOID ARTHRITIS?

Research is being done in many areas, including:

- Immune systems
- Genes
- Families with rheumatoid arthritis
- New drugs or drug combinations
- Rheumatoid arthritis and disability
- Preventing related health problems
- Quality of life for people with rheumatoid arthritis.

Chapter 2: What, Who, How, Why

As stated in Chapter 1, rheumatoid diseases can be very difficult to determine as they take on many different forms. In this chapter we will look closely at various examples of Rheumatic disease.

Osteoarthritis

This is the most common type of arthritis, affecting an estimated 27 million adults in the United States. Osteoarthritis affects both the cartilage, which is the tissue that cushions the ends of bones within the joint, as well as the underlying bone. In osteoarthritis, there is damage to the cartilage, which begins to fray and may wear away entirely. There is also damage to the bond stock of the joint. Osteoarthritis can cause joint pain and stiffness. Disability results most often when the disease affects the spine and the weight-bearing joints (the knees and hips).

Rheumatoid arthritis

This inflammatory disease of the immune system targets first the synovium, or lining of the joint, resulting in pain, stiffness, swelling, joint damage, and loss of function of the joints. Inflammation most often affects joints of the hands and feet and tends to be symmetrical (occurring equally on both sides of the body). This symmetry helps distinguish rheumatoid arthritis from other forms of the disease.

About 0.6 percent of the U.S. population (about 1.3 million people) has rheumatoid arthritis.

Juvenile arthritis

This disease is the most common form of arthritis in childhood, causing pain, stiffness, swelling, and loss of function of the joints. This condition may be associated with rashes or fevers and may affect various parts of the body. Prevalence statistics for juvenile arthritis vary, but about 294,000 children age 0 to 17 are affected with arthritis or other rheumatic conditions.

Fibromyalgia

Fibromyalgia is a chronic disorder that causes pain throughout the tissues that support and move the bones and joints. Pain, stiffness, and localized tender points occur in the muscles and tendons, particularly those of the neck, spine, shoulders, and hips. Patients also may experience fatigue and sleep disturbances. Scientists estimate that fibromyalgia affects 5 million Americans age 18 or older.

Systemic lupus erythematosus

Systemic lupus erythematosus (also known as lupus or SLE) is an autoimmune disease in which the immune system harms the body's own healthy cells and tissues. This can result in inflammation of and damage to the joints, skin, kidneys, heart, lungs, blood vessels, and brain.

Scleroderma

Also known as systemic sclerosis, scleroderma means literally "hard skin." The disease affects the skin, blood vessels, and joints. It may also affect internal organs, such as the lungs and kidneys. In scleroderma, there is an abnormal and excessive production of collagen (a fiber-like protein) in the skin and internal organs.

Spondyloarthropathies

This group of rheumatic diseases principally affects the spine. One common form—ankylosing spondylitis—also may affect the hips, shoulders, and knees. The tendons and ligaments around the bones and joints become inflamed, resulting in pain and stiffness. Ankylosing spondylitis tends to affect people in late adolescence or early adulthood. Reactive arthritis is another spondyloarthropathy. It develops after an infection involving the lower urinary tract, bowel, or other organ. It is commonly associated with eye problems, skin rashes, and mouth sores.

Infectious arthritis

This is a general term used to describe forms of arthritis that are caused by infectious agents, such as bacteria or viruses. Parvovirus arthritis and gonococcal arthritis are examples of infectious arthritis. Arthritis symptoms also may occur in Lyme disease, which is caused by a bacterial infection following the bite of certain ticks. In those cases of arthritis caused by bacteria, early diagnosis and treatment with antibiotics are crucial to removing the infection and minimizing damage to the joints.

Gout

This type of arthritis results from deposits of needle-like crystals of uric acid in the joints. The crystals cause episodic inflammation, swelling, and pain in the affected joint, which is often the big toe. Scientists estimate that 6 million adults age 20 and older report having had gout at some time in their lives.

Polymyalgia rheumatica

Because this disease involves tendons, muscles, ligaments, and tissues around the joint, symptoms often include pain, aching, and morning stiffness in the shoulders, hips, neck, and lower back. It is sometimes the first sign of giant cell arteritis, a disease of the arteries characterized by headaches, inflammation, weakness, weight loss, and fever.

Polymyositis

This rheumatic disease causes inflammation and weakness in the muscles. The disease may affect the whole body and cause disability.

Psoriatic arthritis

This form of arthritis occurs in some patients with psoriasis, a scaling skin disorder. Psoriatic arthritis often affects the joints at the ends of the fingers and toes and is accompanied by changes in the fingernails and toenails. Back pain may occur if the spine is involved.

Bursitis

This condition involves inflammation of the bursae, small, fluid-filled sacs that help reduce friction between bones and other moving structures in the joints. The inflammation may result from arthritis in the joint or injury or infection of the bursae. Bursitis produces pain and tenderness and may limit the movement of nearby joints.

Tendinitis (tendonitis)

This condition refers to inflammation of tendons (tough cords of tissue that connect muscle to bone) caused by overuse, injury, or a rheumatic condition. Tendinitis produces pain and tenderness and may restrict movement of nearby joints.

Now that we have seen some examples of rheumatic diseases, let's move on to understanding the causes of these illnesses.

Rheumatic diseases are generally believed to be caused by a combination of genetic and environmental factors. In other words, you may be born with a susceptibility to a disease, but it may take something in your environment to get the disease started.

Some of these factors have been identified. For example, in osteoarthritis, inherited cartilage weakness or excessive stress on the joint from repeated injury may play a role. In rheumatoid arthritis, juvenile arthritis, and lupus, patients may have a variation in a gene that codes for an enzyme called protein tyrosine phosphatase nonreceptor 22 (PTPN22).

Certain viruses may trigger disease in genetically susceptible people. For example, scientists have found a connection between Epstein-Barr virus and lupus. There are likely many genes and combinations of genes that predispose people to rheumatic diseases, and many different environmental factors that trigger them.

Gender is another factor in some rheumatic diseases. Lupus, rheumatoid arthritis, scleroderma, and fibromyalgia are more common among women. (See next section for details.) This indicates that hormones or other male-female differences may play a role in the development of these conditions.

While rheumatic diseases can affect any individual, there are certain indicators that one can look for.

An estimated 46 million people in the United States have arthritis or other rheumatic conditions.

Rheumatic diseases affect people of all races and ages. Some rheumatic conditions are more common among certain populations. For example:

- Rheumatoid arthritis occurs two to three times more often in women than in men.

- Scleroderma is more common in women than in men.

- Between 80 and 90 percent of those diagnosed with fibromyalgia are women.

- Gout is more common in men than in women. After menopause, the incidence of gout for women begins to rise.

Systemic lupus erythematosus is more common in women than in men, and it occurs more often in African Americans and Hispanics than in Caucasians.

Chapter 3: Signs, Symptoms, Causes and Treatment

Who Has Rheumatoid Arthritis?

Scientists estimate that about 1.3 million people, or about 0.6 percent of the U.S. adult population, have rheumatoid arthritis. Interestingly, some recent studies have suggested that although the number of new cases of rheumatoid arthritis for older people is increasing, the overall number of new cases may actually be going down.

According to the National Arthritis Data Workgroup, the actual number of new cases of rheumatoid arthritis is lower than previous estimates because of changes in the classification for the condition, as cited in Helmick CG, Felson DT, Lawrence RC, Gabriel S, Hirsch R, Kwoh CK, Liang MH, Kremers HM, Mayes MD, Merkel PA, Pillemer SR, Reveille JD, Stone JH, for the National Arthritis Data Workgroup. Estimates of the Prevalence of Arthritis and Other Rheumatic Conditions in the United States. Part I. Arthritis and Rheumatism. 2008;58(1):15-25.

Rheumatoid arthritis occurs in all races and ethnic groups. Although the disease often begins in middle age and occurs with increased frequency in older people, children and young adults also develop it. Like some other forms of arthritis, rheumatoid arthritis occurs much more frequently in women than in men. About two to three times as many women as men have the disease.

What Happens in Rheumatoid Arthritis?

Rheumatoid arthritis is primarily a disease of the joints. A joint is the point where two or more bones come together. With a few exceptions (in the skull and pelvis, for example), joints are designed to allow movement between the bones and to absorb shock from movements like walking or repetitive motions. The ends of the bones are covered by a tough, elastic tissue called cartilage. The joint is surrounded by a capsule that protects and supports it. The joint capsule is lined with a type of tissue called synovium, which produces synovial fluid, a clear substance that lubricates and nourishes the cartilage and bones inside the joint capsule.

Like many other rheumatic diseases, rheumatoid arthritis is an autoimmune disease (*auto* means self), so-called because a person's immune system, which normally helps protect the body from infection and disease, attacks joint tissues for unknown reasons. White blood cells, the agents of the immune system, travel to the synovium and cause inflammation (synovitis), characterized by warmth, redness, swelling, and pain—typical symptoms of rheumatoid arthritis. During the inflammation process, the normally thin synovium becomes thick and makes the joint swollen and puffy to the touch.

As rheumatoid arthritis progresses, the inflamed synovium invades and destroys the cartilage and bone within the joint. The surrounding muscles, ligaments, and tendons that support and stabilize the joint become weak and unable to work normally. These effects lead to the pain and joint damage often seen in rheumatoid arthritis. Researchers studying rheumatoid arthritis now believe that it begins to damage bones during the first year or two that a person has the disease, one reason why early diagnosis and treatment are so important.

Some people with rheumatoid arthritis also have symptoms in places other than their joints. Many people with rheumatoid arthritis develop anemia, or a decrease in the production of red blood cells. Other effects that occur less often include neck pain and dry eyes and mouth. Very rarely, people may have inflammation of the blood vessels (vasculitis), the lining of the lungs (pleurisy), or the sac enclosing the heart (pericarditis).

A joint (the place where two bones meet) is surrounded by a capsule that protects and supports it. The joint capsule is lined with a type of tissue called synovium, which produces synovial fluid that lubricates and nourishes joint tissues. In rheumatoid arthritis, the synovium becomes inflamed, causing warmth, redness, swelling, and pain. As the disease progresses, the inflamed synovium invades and damages the cartilage and bone of the joint. Surrounding muscles, ligaments, and tendons become weakened. Rheumatoid arthritis also can cause more generalized bone loss that may lead to osteoporosis (fragile bones that are prone to fracture).

How Does Rheumatoid Arthritis Affect People's Lives?

Rheumatoid arthritis affects people differently. For some people, it lasts only a few months or a year or two and goes away without causing any noticeable damage. Other people have mild or moderate forms of the disease, with periods of worsening symptoms, called flares, and periods in which they feel better, called remissions. Still others have a severe form of the disease that is active most of the time, lasts for many years or a lifetime, and leads to serious joint damage and disability.

Although rheumatoid arthritis is primarily a disease of the joints, its effects are not just physical. Many people with rheumatoid arthritis also experience issues related to:

- depression, anxiety
- feelings of helplessness
- low self-esteem.

Rheumatoid arthritis can affect virtually every area of a person's life from work life to family life. One study showed that more than a quarter of women stopped working within 4 years after being diagnosed with rheumatoid arthritis. Rheumatoid arthritis can also interfere with the joys and responsibilities of family life and may affect the decision to have children.

Fortunately, current treatment strategies, including pain-relieving drugs and medications that slow joint damage, a balance between rest and exercise, and patient education and support programs, allow most people with the disease to lead active and productive lives. In recent years, research has led to a new understanding of rheumatoid arthritis and has increased the likelihood that, in time, researchers will find even better ways to treat the disease.

What Causes Rheumatoid Arthritis?

Scientists still do not know exactly what causes the immune system to turn against itself in rheumatoid arthritis, but research over the last few years has begun to piece together the factors involved.

Genetic (inherited) factors: Scientists have discovered that certain genes known to play a role in the immune system are associated with a tendency to develop rheumatoid arthritis. For the genes that have been linked to rheumatoid arthritis, the frequency of the risky gene is only modestly higher in those with rheumatoid arthritis compared with healthy controls. In other words, individual genes by themselves confer only a small relative risk of disease. Some people who have these particular genes never develop the disease. These observations suggest that although a person's genetic makeup plays an important role in determining if he or she will develop rheumatoid arthritis, it is not the only factor. What is clear, however, is that more than one gene is involved in determining whether a person develops rheumatoid arthritis and how severe the disease will become.

Environmental factors: Many scientists think that something must occur to trigger the disease process in people whose genetic makeup makes them susceptible to rheumatoid arthritis. A viral or bacterial infection appears likely, but the exact agent is not yet known. This does not mean that rheumatoid arthritis is contagious: a person cannot catch it from someone else.

Other factors: Some scientists also think that a variety of hormonal factors may be involved. Women are more likely to develop rheumatoid arthritis than men. The disease may improve during pregnancy and flare after pregnancy.

Breastfeeding may also aggravate the disease. Contraceptive use may alter a person's likelihood of developing rheumatoid arthritis. This suggests hormones, or possibly deficiencies or changes in certain hormones, may promote the development of rheumatoid arthritis in a genetically susceptible person who has been exposed to a triggering agent from the environment.

Even though all the answers are not known, one thing is certain: rheumatoid arthritis develops as a result of an interaction of many factors. Researchers are trying to understand these factors and how they work together.

How Is Rheumatoid Arthritis Diagnosed?

Rheumatoid arthritis can be difficult to diagnose in its early stages for several reasons. First, there is no single test for the disease. In addition, symptoms differ from person to person and can be more severe in some people than in others. Also, symptoms can be similar to those of other types of arthritis and joint conditions, and it may take some time for other conditions to be ruled out. Finally, the full range of symptoms develops over time, and only a few symptoms may be present in the early stages. As a result, doctors use a variety of the following tools to diagnose the disease and to rule out other conditions:

Medical history: The doctor begins by asking the patient to describe the symptoms, and when and how the condition started, as well as how the symptoms have changed over time. The doctor will also ask about any other medical problems the patient and close family members have and about any medications the patient is taking. Accurate answers to these questions can help the doctor make a diagnosis and understand the impact the disease has on the patient's life.

Good communication between patient and doctor is especially important. For example, the patient's description of pain, stiffness, and joint function and how these change over time is critical to the doctor's initial assessment of the disease and how it changes over time.

Physical examination: The doctor will check the patient's reflexes and general health, including muscle strength. The doctor will also examine bothersome joints and observe the patient's ability to walk, bend, and carry out activities of daily living. The doctor will also look at the skin for a rash and listen to the chest for signs of inflammation in the lungs.

Laboratory tests: A number of lab tests may be useful in confirming a diagnosis of rheumatoid arthritis. Following are some of the more common ones:

Rheumatoid factor (RF): Rheumatoid factor is an antibody that is present eventually in the blood of most people with rheumatoid arthritis. (An antibody is a special protein made by the immune system that normally helps fight foreign substances in the body.) Not all people with rheumatoid arthritis test positive for rheumatoid factor, and some people test positive for rheumatoid factor, yet never develop the disease. Rheumatoid factor also can be positive in some other diseases; however, a positive RF in a person who has symptoms consistent with those of rheumatoid arthritis can be useful in confirming a diagnosis. Furthermore, high levels of rheumatoid factor are associated with more severe rheumatoid arthritis.

Anti-CCP antibodies: This blood test detects antibodies to cyclic citrullinated peptide (anti-CCP). This test is positive in most people with rheumatoid arthritis and can even be positive years before rheumatoid arthritis symptoms develop. When used with the RF, this test's results are very useful in confirming a rheumatoid arthritis diagnosis.

Others: Other common laboratory tests include a white blood cell count, a blood test for anemia, which is common in rheumatoid arthritis; the erythrocyte sedimentation rate (often called the sed rate), which measures inflammation in the body; and C-reactive protein, another common test for inflammation that is useful both in making a diagnosis and monitoring disease activity and response to anti-inflammatory therapy.

X rays: X rays are used to determine the degree of joint destruction. They are not useful in the early stages of rheumatoid arthritis before bone damage is evident; however, they may be used to rule out other causes of joint pain. They may also be used later to monitor the progression of the disease.

How Is Rheumatoid Arthritis Treated?

Doctors use a variety of approaches to treat rheumatoid arthritis. These are used in different combinations and at different times during the course of the disease and are chosen according to the patient's individual situation. No matter what treatment the doctor and patient choose, however, the goals are the same: to relieve pain, reduce inflammation, slow down or stop joint damage, and improve the person's sense of well-being and ability to function.

Good communication between the patient and doctor is necessary for effective treatment. Talking to the doctor can help ensure that exercise and pain management programs are provided as needed, and that drugs are prescribed appropriately. Talking to the doctor can also help people who are making decisions about surgery.

Goals of Treatment

- Relieve pain

- Reduce inflammation

- Slow down or stop joint damage

- Improve a person's sense of well-being and ability to function.

Current Treatment Approaches

- Lifestyle

- Medications

- Surgery

- Routine monitoring and ongoing care.

Health behavior changes: Certain activities can help improve a person's ability to function independently and maintain a positive outlook.

Rest and exercise: People with rheumatoid arthritis need a good balance between rest and exercise, with more rest when the disease is active and more exercise when it is not. Rest helps to reduce active joint inflammation and pain and to fight fatigue. The length of time for rest will vary from person to person, but in general, shorter rest breaks every now and then are more helpful than long times spent in bed.

Exercise is important for maintaining healthy and strong muscles, preserving joint mobility, and maintaining flexibility. Exercise can also help people sleep well, reduce pain, maintain a positive attitude, and lose weight. Exercise programs should take into account the person's physical abilities, limitations, and changing needs.

Joint care: Some people find using a splint for a short time around a painful joint reduces pain and swelling by supporting the joint and letting it rest. Splints are used mostly on wrists and hands, but also on ankles and feet. A doctor or a physical or occupational therapist can help a person choose a splint and make sure it fits properly. Other ways to reduce stress on joints include self-help devices (for example, zipper pullers, long-handled shoe horns); devices to help with getting on and off chairs, toilet seats, and beds; and changes in the ways that a person carries out daily activities.

Stress reduction: People with rheumatoid arthritis face emotional challenges as well as physical ones. The emotions they feel because of the disease—fear, anger, and frustration—combined with any pain and physical limitations can increase their stress level. Although there is no evidence that stress plays a role in causing rheumatoid arthritis, it can make living with the disease difficult at times. Stress also may affect the amount of pain a person feels. There are a number of successful techniques for coping with stress. Regular rest periods can help, as can relaxation, distraction, or visualization exercises. Exercise programs, participation in support groups, and good communication with the health care team are other ways to reduce stress.

Healthful diet: With the exception of several specific types of oils, there is no scientific evidence that any specific food or nutrient helps or harms people with rheumatoid arthritis. However, an overall nutritious diet with enough—but not an excess of—calories, protein, and calcium is important. Some people may need to be careful about drinking alcoholic beverages because of the medications they take for rheumatoid arthritis. Those taking methotrexate may need to avoid alcohol altogether because one of the most serious long-term side effects of methotrexate is liver damage.

Climate: Some people notice that their arthritis gets worse when there is a sudden change in the weather. However, there is no evidence that a specific climate can prevent or reduce the effects of rheumatoid arthritis. Moving to a new place with a different climate usually does not make a long-term difference in a person's rheumatoid arthritis.

Medications: Most people who have rheumatoid arthritis take medications. Some medications (analgesics) are used only for pain relief; others [corticosteroids and nonsteroidal anti-inflammatory drugs (NSAIDs)] are used to reduce inflammation. Still others, often called disease-modifying antirheumatic drugs (DMARDs), are used to try to slow the course of the disease. The newest and perhaps most promising class of arthritis medications are the biologic response modifiers. These are genetically engineered medications that help reduce inflammation and structural damage to the joints by interrupting the cascade of events that drive inflammation. Currently, seven biologic response modifiers are approved for rheumatoid arthritis. They work in one of several ways:

- Four of these drugs, etanercept (Enbrel), golimumab (Simponi), infliximab (Remicade), and adalimumab (Humira), reduce inflammation by blocking tumor necrosis factor (TNF), a cytokine or immune system protein that triggers inflammation during normal immune responses.

- Anakinra (Kineret), works by blocking a cytokine called interleukin-1 (IL-1) that is seen in excess in patients with rheumatoid arthritis.

- Rituximab (Rituxan) stops the activation of a type of white blood cell called B cells. This reduces the overall activity of the immune system, which is overactive in people with rheumatoid arthritis.

- Abatacept (Orencia) blocks a particular chemical that triggers the overproduction of white blood cells called T cells that play a role in rheumatoid arthritis inflammation.

[2]Brand names included in this booklet are provided as examples only, and their inclusion does not mean that these products are endorsed by the National Institutes of Health or any other Government agency. Also, if a particular brand name is not mentioned, this does not mean or imply that the product is unsatisfactory.

For many years, doctors initially prescribed aspirin or other pain-relieving drugs for rheumatoid arthritis, and waited to prescribe more powerful drugs only if the disease worsened.

In recent decades this approach to treatment has changed as studies have shown that early treatment with more powerful drugs—and the use of drug combinations instead of one medication alone—may be more effective in reducing or preventing joint damage. Someone with persistent rheumatoid arthritis symptoms should see a doctor familiar with the disease and its treatment to reduce the risk of damage.

The person's general condition, the current and predicted severity of the illness, the length of time he or she will take the drug, and the drug's effectiveness and potential side effects are important considerations in prescribing drugs for rheumatoid arthritis. Many of the new drugs that help reduce disease in rheumatoid arthritis do so by reducing the inflammation that can cause pain and joint damage. However, in some instances, inflammation is one mechanism the body normally uses to maintain health, such as to fight infection and possibly to stop tumors from growing. The magnitude of the risk from the treatment is hard to judge because infections and cancer can occur in patients with rheumatoid arthritis who are not on treatment, and probably more commonly than in healthy individuals. Nevertheless, appropriate caution and vigilance are justified.

Surgery: Several types of surgery are available to patients with severe joint damage. The primary purpose of these procedures is to reduce pain, improve the affected joint's function, and improve the patient's ability to perform daily activities. Surgery is not for everyone, however, and the decision should be made only after careful consideration by the patient and doctor. Together they should discuss the patient's overall health, the condition of the joint or tendon that will be operated on, and the reason for, as well as the risks and benefits of, the surgical procedure. Cost may be another factor.

Following are some of the more common surgeries performed for rheumatoid arthritis:

Joint replacement: Joint replacement involves removing all or part of a damaged joint and replacing it with synthetic components. Joint replacement is available for a number of different joints, but the most commonly replaced joints are the hips and knees. Joint replacement surgery is done primarily to relieve pain and improve or preserve function.

Although joint replacement traditionally involved a large incision and long recovery, new minimally invasive surgeries are making it possible to do some forms of joint replacement with smaller incisions and a shorter, easier recovery.

Artificial joints are not always permanent and may eventually have to be replaced. This may be an important consideration for young people.

Arthrodesis (fusion): Arthrodesis is a surgical procedure that involves removing the joint and fusing the bones into one immobile unit, often using bone grafts from the person's own pelvis. Although the procedure limits movement, it can be useful for increasing stability and relieving pain in affected joints. The most commonly fused joints are the ankles and wrists and joints of the fingers and toes.

Tendon reconstruction: Rheumatoid arthritis can damage and even rupture tendons, the tissues that attach muscle to bone. This surgery, which is used most frequently on the hands, reconstructs the damaged tendon by attaching an intact tendon to it. This procedure can help to restore hand function, especially if the tendon is completely ruptured.

Synovectomy: In this surgery, the doctor actually removes the inflamed synovial tissue. Synovectomy by itself is seldom performed now because not all of the tissue can be removed, and it eventually grows back. Synovectomy is done as part of reconstructive surgery, especially tendon reconstruction.

Routine monitoring and ongoing care: Regular medical care is important to monitor the course of the disease, determine the effectiveness and any negative effects of medications, and change therapies as needed.

Monitoring typically includes regular visits to the doctor. It also may include blood, urine, and other laboratory tests and x rays.

People with rheumatoid arthritis may want to discuss preventing osteoporosis with their doctors as part of their long-term, ongoing care. Osteoporosis is a condition in which bones become weakened and fragile. Having rheumatoid arthritis increases the risk of developing osteoporosis for both men and women, particularly if a person takes corticosteroids. Such patients may want to discuss with their doctors the potential benefits of calcium and vitamin D supplements or other treatments for osteoporosis.

Alternative and complementary therapies: Special diets, vitamin supplements, and other alternative approaches have been suggested for treating rheumatoid arthritis.

Research shows that some of these, for example, fish oil supplements, may help reduce arthritis inflammation. For most, however, controlled scientific studies either have not been conducted on them or have found no definite benefit to these therapies.

As with any therapy, patients should discuss the benefits and drawbacks with their doctors before beginning an alternative or new type of therapy. If the doctor feels the approach has value and will not be harmful, it can be incorporated into a patient's treatment plan. However, it is important not to neglect regular health care. The Arthritis Foundation publishes material on alternative therapies as well as established therapies, and patients may want to contact this organization for information.

Who Treats Rheumatoid Arthritis?

Diagnosing and treating rheumatoid arthritis requires a team effort involving the patient and several types of health care professionals.

The primary doctor to treat arthritis may be an **internist**, a doctor who specializes in the diagnosis and medical treatment of adults, or a **rheumatologist**, a doctor who specializes in arthritis and other diseases of the bones, joints, and muscles.

As treatment progresses, other professionals often help. These may include the following:

Orthopaedists: Surgeons who specialize in the treatment of, and surgery for, bone and joint diseases.

Physical therapists: Health professionals who work with patients to improve joint function.

Occupational therapists: Health professionals who teach ways to protect joints, minimize pain, perform activities of daily living, and conserve energy.

Dietitians: Health professionals who teach ways to use a good diet to improve health and maintain a healthy weight.

Nurse educators: Nurses who specialize in helping patients understand their overall condition and implement their treatment plans.

Psychologists: Health professionals who seek to help patients cope with difficulties in the home and workplace that may result from their medical conditions.

Chapter 4: What You Can Do!

The Importance of Self-Care

Although health care professionals can prescribe or recommend treatments to help patients manage their rheumatoid arthritis, the real key to living well with the disease are the patients themselves. Research shows that people who take part in their own care report less pain and make fewer doctor visits. They also enjoy a better quality of life.

Patient education and arthritis self-management programs, as well as support groups, help people to become better informed and to participate in their own care. An example of a self-management program is the Arthritis Self-Help Course offered by the Arthritis Foundation and developed at a NIAMS-supported Multipurpose Arthritis and Musculoskeletal Diseases Center. (See the Arthritis Foundation listing in "For More Information.") Self-management programs teach about rheumatoid arthritis and its treatments, exercise and relaxation approaches, communication between patients and health care providers, and problem solving. Research on these programs has shown that they help people:

- understand the disease

- reduce their pain while remaining active

- cope physically, emotionally, and mentally

- feel greater control over the disease and build a sense of confidence in the ability to function and lead full, active, and independent lives.

Healty Diets

Special diets, vitamin supplements, and other alternative approaches have been suggested for treating rheumatoid arthritis. Although such approaches may not be harmful, scientific studies have not yet shown any benefits.

An overall nutritious diet with the right amount of calories, protein, and calcium is important. Some people need to be careful about drinking alcoholic beverages because of the medications they take for rheumatoid arthritis.

Scientists are making rapid progress in understanding the complexities of rheumatoid arthritis. They are learning more about how and why it develops and why some people have more severe symptoms than others.

Preventing Related Problems

Having rheumatoid arthritis does not make people immune to other medical problems. Thus, reducing the risk of problems that can be associated with rheumatoid arthritis is a focus of NIAMS research. One recent study showed that treatment with hydroxychloroquine, a medication used to treat rheumatic diseases and malaria, reduced the incidence of diabetes in people with rheumatoid arthritis. People with rheumatoid arthritis who took the medication for more than 4 years showed a reduction in risk of diabetes of up to 77 percent.

Hope for the Future

Scientists are making rapid progress in understanding the complexities of rheumatoid arthritis: how and why it develops, why some people get it and others do not, why some people get it more severely than others. Results from research are having an impact today, enabling people with rheumatoid arthritis to remain active in life, family, and work far longer than was possible 20 years ago. There is also hope for tomorrow, as researchers begin to apply new technologies such as stem cell transplantation and novel imaging techniques. (Stem cells have the capacity to differentiate into specific cell types, which gives them the potential to change damaged tissue in which they are placed.) These and other advances will lead to an improved quality of life for people with rheumatoid arthritis.

Chapter 5: Key Terms and Ongoing Research

What Research Is Being Done on Rheumatoid Arthritis?

Over the last several decades, research has greatly increased our understanding of the immune system, genetics, and biology. This research is now showing results in several areas important to rheumatoid arthritis. Scientists are thinking about rheumatoid arthritis in exciting ways that were not possible even 10 years ago.

The National Institutes of Health (NIH) funds a wide variety of medical research at its headquarters in Bethesda, MD, and at universities and medical centers across the United States. One of the NIH institutes, the National Institute of Arthritis and Musculoskeletal and Skin Diseases (NIAMS), is a major supporter of research and research training in rheumatoid arthritis through grants to individual scientists, Specialized Centers of Research, Multidisciplinary Clinical Research Centers, and Multipurpose Arthritis and Musculoskeletal Diseases Centers.

Following are examples of current research directions in rheumatoid arthritis.

Genetics

Researchers are studying genetic factors that predispose some people to developing rheumatoid arthritis, as well as factors connected with disease severity. In recent years, NIAMS-supported research in this area has led to several important genetic discoveries including the following:

Variation in a gene involved in controlling T-cell activation doubles rheumatoid arthritis risk: The variation—called a single nucleotide polymorphism (SNP)—is located within a gene that codes for PTPN22, an enzyme known to be involved in controlling the activation of white blood cells called T cells that play an important role in the body's immune system. Where the SNP is present in one or both copies of a person's genes for this enzyme, T cells and other immune cells respond too vigorously, causing increased inflammation and tissue damage. Scientists say the implications of this finding go beyond a better understanding of rheumatoid arthritis risk; it may also help explain why different autoimmune diseases tend to run in families. Other studies have the same SNP with type-1 diabetes and juvenile arthritis.

Genetic variation increases risk of rheumatoid arthritis and lupus: Separate research found a SNP in a large segment of the STAT4 gene increases the risk of both rheumatoid arthritis and another autoimmune disease, systemic lupus erythematosus (lupus). The STAT4 gene encodes a protein that plays an important role in the regulation and activation of certain cells of the immune system. One variant form of the gene was present at a significantly higher frequency in rheumatoid arthritis patient samples from the North American Rheumatoid Arthritis Consortium (NARAC)—a consortium formed to collect, analyze, and make available clinical and genetic data on 1,000 sibling pairs with rheumatoid arthritis—as compared with controls. Scientists replicated that result in two independent collections of rheumatoid arthritis cases and controls.

Twin study shows genetic differences in rheumatoid arthritis: Because identical twins have the exact same genes at conception, scientists believe that changes in the genes after the genome is constructed may account for why one of a twin pair can have rheumatoid arthritis while the other does not. To better understand what those changes might be, scientists have used a sophisticated technique called microarray to examine the expression of more than 20,000 genes at a time in 11 pairs of disease-discordant identical twins (meaning one twin had the disease, the other did not). The examination led to the detection of differences in expression of 827 genes. The most significantly overexpressed gene was laeverin, an enzyme that breaks down certain types of proteins; second was 11ß-hydroxysteroid dehydrogenase type 2 (11ß-HSD2), important in a steroid pathway linked to inflammation and bone erosion; and third was cysteine-rich angiogenic inducer 61 (Cyr61), which is known for its role in angiogenesis, the formation of new blood vessels. The scientists say their findings are exciting because they offer new insights into the mechanisms by which rheumatoid arthritis is mediated.

Genetic region associated with rheumatoid arthritis risk: Using the relatively new genome-wide association approach, which makes it possible to analyze between 300,000 and 500,000 single nucleotide polymorphisms, researchers in the United States and Sweden identified a region of chromosome 9 containing two genes relevant to chronic inflammation: TRAF1 (encoding tumor necrosis factor receptor-associated factor 1) and C5 (encoding complement component 5). Scientists say it is not yet known how the genes in the TRAF1-C5 region influence rheumatoid arthritis risk, but they hope that by learning more about the genes and their role in the disease, they may find clues to influencing treatment of the disease.

Rheumatoid Arthritis and Disability

During the past 20 years, significant changes in managing rheumatoid arthritis, including new and more powerful drugs and more aggressive treatment, have improved both shortand long-term disability outcomes. Using data from 3,035 patients enrolled in the ARAMIS (Arthritis, Rheumatism, and Aging Medical Information System) data bank—a large data bank with treatment history for a broad range of patients, and containing widely accepted disability measurements—NIAMS-supported researchers found that average disability levels in patients with rheumatoid arthritis have declined by 40 percent since 1977 at a rate of about 2 percent a year.

Despite recent improvements in treatment and disability outcomes, women with rheumatoid arthritis may have difficulty maintaining jobs, one NIAMS-supported study shows. Researchers who followed two groups of women with rheumatoid arthritis 11 years apart—the first group beginning in 1987, the second in 1998—found the rate at which women left the workforce did not fall significantly. They found that more than a quarter of the women in both groups stopped working within 4 years after being diagnosed with rheumatoid arthritis.

Researchers cited several possible reasons to explain why the rate of stopping work did not decline, even while disease activity did. They concluded that patients' reasons for leaving work had changed between the time the 1987 and 1998 groups were studied, and that more women were leaving work in 1998 for reasons other than increased disease activity.

Potential Treatments

Researchers continue to identify molecules that appear to play a role in rheumatoid arthritis and thus are potential targets for new treatments. The path between identifying the molecule and developing a drug that targets it is long and difficult. Fortunately, this path has been successfully negotiated and new drugs have emerged that successfully reduce symptoms and damage in rheumatoid arthritis. Researchers continue to identify more candidate drugs, with hopes that these will have fewer side effects or will cure more patients.

Understanding Joint Destruction

Advances in understanding the processes that lead to joint destruction are bringing NIAMS-supported researchers a step closer to new therapies to stop the destructive process. In one NIAMS study researchers found a factor they suspect plays a crucial role in joint destruction: an adhesion molecule on cells of the synovium called cadherin-11. Adhesion molecules allow individual cells to stick together to form tissues. At normal levels, cadherin-11 enables the cells (synoviocytes) to adhere together to form the lining layer of the synovium. But when overgrowth of the synovium occurs, cadherin plays a key role in the destructive behavior of the synovium; namely, eroding the cartilage, which causes permanent destruction to the joint. In studies of mice prone to a disease similar to human rheumatoid arthritis, blocking cadherin-11 prevented cartilage destruction. The next step is to determine whether an agent to block an excess of the molecule has the same beneficial effect in people with rheumatoid arthritis.

In other research scientists found that a lack of apoptosis (programmed cell death) contributes to a proliferation of cells in the joint lining and the failure to eliminate immune cells that react against self. In animal studies, mice lacking two proteins that mediate the process of apoptosis developed arthritis.

Key Words

Analgesics. Medications designed to relieve pain. Pure analgesics do not have an effect on inflammation.

Anti-CCP antibodies. Antibodies to cyclic citrullinated peptide (anti-CCP). A positive test for the antibodies is useful for confirming a diagnosis of rheumatoid arthritis. In fact, tests for the antibodies can be positive years before the development of symptoms.

Apoptosis. Programmed cell death. This is a mechanism by which the body rids itself of old or unhealthy cells. A problem with this mechanism can allow cells that react against the body's own tissues to survive.

Arthrodesis. A surgical procedure that involves removing the joint and fusing the bones into one immobile unit, often using bone grafts from the person's own pelvis. Although the procedure limits movement, it can be useful for increasing stability and relieving pain in affected joints. The most commonly fused joints are the ankles and wrists and joints of the fingers and toes.

Autoimmune disease. A disease in which the immune system, which is designed to protect the body from foreign invaders, mistakenly sees the body's own tissues as foreign and makes autoantibodies against them, leading to tissue destruction.

Biologic response modifiers. Genetically engineered medications that help reduce inflammation and structural damage to the joints by interrupting the cascade of events that drive inflammation.

C-reactive protein. A protein produced by the body during the process of inflammation. A positive blood test for the protein indicates the presence of inflammation in the body. The test may be used in diagnosing rheumatoid arthritis and monitoring disease activity and the response of treatment.

Cartilage. A tough, elastic tissue that covers the ends of the bones where they meet to form joints. In rheumatoid arthritis, the inflamed synovium invades and destroys joint cartilage.

Collagen. A family of fibrous proteins that are components of cartilage. Collagens are the building blocks of skin, tendon, bone, and other connective tissues.

Corticosteroids. Powerful anti-inflammatory hormones made naturally in the body or man made for use as medicine. Corticosteroids may be taken orally to relieve the systemic inflammation of rheumatoid arthritis or injected directly into an inflamed joint to temporarily reduce inflammation and relieve pain.

COX-2 inhibitors. A subclass of nonsteroidal anti-inflammatory drugs (NSAIDs) that are formulated to relieve pain and inflammation with less risk of gastrointestinal ulcers.

Diabetes. A disease that affects the body's ability to produce or use insulin, resulting in an inability to control the level of sugar in the blood. If not properly treated, high blood sugar levels can eventually lead to problems such as kidney disease, heart disease, and blindness.

Dietitian. A health professional who teaches ways to use a good diet to improve health and maintain a healthy weight.

Disease-modifying antirheumatic drugs (DMARDs). A class of medications used in the treatment of rheumatoid arthritis. DMARDs do more than ease the symptoms of rheumatoid arthritis like some other treatments. They often slow or stop the course of the disease to help prevent joint damage.

Erythrocyte sedimentation rate (sed rate). A blood test used to detect and monitor inflammation. It is measured by recording the rate at which red blood cells fall and form sediment at the bottom of a test tube.

Flare. A period of heightened disease activity. In rheumatoid arthritis, a flare may be characterized by increased fatigue; fever; and painful, swollen, and tender joints.

Hydroxychloroquine. An anti-inflammatory drug used in the treatment of rheumatoid arthritis, malaria, and lupus.

Immune system. A complex network of cells and tissues that work in concert to protect the body against invaders such as viruses and bacteria.

Joint capsule. A tough membrane sac that holds the bones and other joint parts together.

Ligaments. Tough bands of connective tissue that attach bones to each other, providing stability.

Lupus. A chronic inflammatory condition in which the immune system attacks the skin, joints, heart, lungs, blood, kidneys and brain. Also called systemic lupus erythematosus.

Muscles. Bundles of specialized cells that contract and relax to produce movement when stimulated by nerves.

Nonsteroidal anti-inflammatory drugs (NSAIDs). A class of medications available over the counter or with a prescription that ease pain and inflammation. Commonly used NSAIDs include ibuprofen (Advil, Motrin), naproxen sodium (Aleve), and ketoprofen (Orudis, Oruvail).

Nurse educator. A nurse who specializes in helping patients understand their overall condition and implementing their treatment plans.

Occupational therapist. A health professional who teaches ways to protect joints, minimize pain, perform activities of daily living, and conserve energy.

Orthopaedist. A surgeon who specializes in the treatment of, and surgery for, bone and joint diseases. Also called orthopaedic surgeon.

Pericarditis. Inflammation of the pericardium, the thin sac-like membrane that surrounds the heart. Pericarditis can be caused by rheumatoid arthritis.

Physical therapist. A health professional who works with patients to improve joint function.

Pleurisy. Inflammation of the pleura, the linings surrounding the lungs. Pleurisy can be caused by rheumatoid arthritis.

Psychologist. A health professional who seeks to help patients cope with difficulties in the home and workplace that may result from their medical conditions.

Rheumatoid arthritis. A form of arthritis in which the immune system attacks the tissues of the joints, leading to pain, inflammation, and eventually joint damage and malformation. It causes swelling and redness in joints, and may make people feel sick, tired, and feverish. Rheumatoid arthritis may also affect skin tissue, the lungs, the eyes, or the blood vessels.

Rheumatoid factor (RF). An antibody that is present eventually in the blood of most people with rheumatoid arthritis. Not all people with rheumatoid arthritis test positive for rheumatoid factor, and some people test positive for rheumatoid factor, yet never develop the disease. Rheumatoid factor also can be positive in some other diseases.

Synovectomy. Removal of the synovium (joint lining). As a treatment for rheumatoid arthritis, synovectomy is much less common than it once was because not all of the tissue can be removed, and it eventually grows back. Synovectomy is done as part of reconstructive surgery, especially tendon reconstruction.

Synovium. A thin membrane inside the joint capsule that secretes synovial fluid. In rheumatoid arthritis, the synovium is attacked by the immune system.

Synovial fluid. A fluid secreted by the synovium that lubricates the joint and keeps the cartilage smooth and healthy.

Tendons. Tough, fibrous cords that connect muscles to bones.

Vasculitis. Inflammation of the blood vessels. Vasculitis can occur as a complication of rheumatoid arthritis.

X ray. A procedure in which low-level radiation is passed through the body to produce a picture called a radiograph. X rays of joints affected by rheumatoid arthritis are used to determine the degree of joint destruction.

www.MedicalCenter.com

Printed in Great Britain
by Amazon

39557730R10026